AIP

DIET

For

HASIMOTO'S

Hasimoto's AIP CookBook with Recipes and meal plans for the diagnosed

Copyright © 2023 by Sarah Thompson

All rights reserved

This copyrights page explains the legal rights and protections related to the content of this nonfiction book for readers and users. You understand that you have the right to access or use this book in any way, including reading, downloading, or sharing. Ownership and Intellectual Property Rights: The content, graphics, and other elements in this nonfiction book are all covered by copyright and other intellectual property laws. Sarah Thompson is the only owner of the content. Any unauthorized use or reproduction of this book's content may be illegal and give rise to legal action. For reading and using this book for personal, non-commercial uses only, you have been granted a constrained, non-exclusive, and non-transferable permission. You are prohibited from altering, distributing or Without Sarah Thompson's prior written approval, you may not distribute, communicate, display, perform, reproduce, publish, license, create derivative works from, transfer, or sell any portion of the book.

TABLE OF CONTENTS

ONE POT MEAL PLAN

COMFORT FOOD MEAL PLAN

1

RECOVERING FROM HASHIMOTO'S WITH THE AUTOIMMUNE PROTOCOL (AIP)

Hashimoto's thyroiditis is an autoimmune disorder that affects the thyroid gland, leading to an underactive thyroid (hypothyroidism). The condition is characterized by the immune system mistakenly attacking the thyroid tissue, causing inflammation and disruption in thyroid hormone production. One approach gaining attention for managing Hashimoto's is the Autoimmune Protocol (AIP), a specialized diet and lifestyle regimen designed to reduce inflammation, heal the gut, and potentially alleviate autoimmune symptoms.

The Autoimmune Protocol is an extension of the paleo diet, focusing on nutrient-dense, whole foods while eliminating potential triggers that can exacerbate autoimmune responses. The core principles of AIP include removing foods like grains, legumes, dairy, refined sugars, processed foods, and nightshade vegetables, as these items are believed to contribute to inflammation and gut dysfunction, which are often implicated in autoimmune conditions like Hashimoto's.

Central to the AIP is its emphasis on gut health. Research suggests that there is a strong connection between gut health and autoimmune disorders, including Hashimoto's. The AIP diet aims to repair the intestinal lining, which may have become permeable (leaky gut) due to inflammation and other factors. By consuming nutrient-rich foods like bone broth, fermented vegetables, and healthy fats, individuals following AIP can support gut healing and restoration.

Another important aspect of the AIP approach is its focus on reducing inflammation. Chronic inflammation is a hallmark of autoimmune diseases, and certain foods can exacerbate this process. By eliminating inflammatory foods and incorporating anti-inflammatory choices like fatty fish, turmeric, and berries, individuals with Hashimoto's may experience a reduction in overall inflammation, potentially leading to improved thyroid function and symptom management.

Additionally, AIP encourages adequate sleep, stress management, regular exercise, and mindfulness practices. These lifestyle factors are crucial in supporting the immune system, reducing stress-related triggers, and promoting overall well-being. Stress, in particular, has been linked to autoimmune flares, so practicing relaxation techniques and adopting stress-reduction strategies can be immensely beneficial for those on the path to Hashimoto's recovery.

It's important to note that the Autoimmune Protocol is not a one-size-fits-all solution. Each person's experience with Hashimoto's is unique, and while AIP has shown promise for many individuals, consulting with a healthcare professional before making any significant dietary or lifestyle changes is essential. Monitoring thyroid function and working closely with a knowledgeable healthcare provider can ensure that the AIP approach is tailored to an individual's specific needs and health goals.

Recovering from Hashimoto's with the Autoimmune Protocol involves a comprehensive approach that encompasses dietary adjustments, gut healing, inflammation reduction, and mindful lifestyle practices. By adhering to the principles of AIP and working in collaboration with healthcare experts, individuals with Hashimoto's have the potential to take an active role in managing their condition and promoting overall wellness.

Supplements and Nutritional Support:

Navigating the intricacies of the Autoimmune Protocol (AIP) can be both rewarding and challenging for individuals seeking to manage autoimmune conditions through dietary means. While the AIP diet focuses on eliminating potential trigger foods to alleviate inflammation and promote healing, ensuring proper nutritional support is crucial to maintain overall health and well-being. In many cases, achieving all essential nutrients solely through diet can be complex, leading to the consideration of supplements as a means of enhancing the AIP journey.

Supplements can play a supportive role in addressing potential nutrient deficiencies, supporting immune function, and optimizing overall health for AIP patients. However, it's important to approach supplementation with careful consideration, as not all supplements are suitable for the AIP framework. Collaborating with a healthcare professional who is knowledgeable about the AIP diet and its unique requirements is recommended before introducing supplements into the regimen.

In this exploration of supplements and nutritional support for AIP patients, we will delve into key nutrients commonly emphasized in the AIP diet, discuss potential deficiencies, and highlight supplements that align with AIP principles. Remember, while supplements can be valuable tools, they should complement a well-rounded AIP-compliant diet and not replace the foundation of nutrient-rich foods that forms the basis of the healing journey.

ESSENTIAL NUTRIENTS FOR HASHIMOTO'S RECOVERY

Embarking on the journey to overcome Hashimoto's thyroiditis through the Autoimmune Protocol (AIP) demands a comprehensive approach, one that extends beyond mere dietary restrictions. AIP, a therapeutic framework designed to alleviate inflammation and restore immune balance, is a beacon of hope for those grappling with this autoimmune thyroid condition. Central to this approach is a keen focus on consuming essential nutrients that not only support overall health but also play a pivotal role in Hashimoto's recovery.

In the pursuit of vitality and healing, it becomes evident that Hashimoto's thyroiditis not only affects the thyroid but reverberates through various bodily systems. By harnessing the power of nutrient-dense foods, AIP patients can supply their bodies with the building blocks required for cellular rejuvenation, immune modulation, and hormonal equilibrium. From vitamins and minerals that bolster immunity to antioxidants that combat oxidative stress, each nutrient plays a distinct role in the intricate dance of Hashimoto's healing.

In this exploration of essential nutrients for Hashimoto's recovery within the context of the AIP framework, we will delve into the profound impact of specific vitamins, minerals, and antioxidants. From selenium's thyroid-supportive prowess to the inflammation-taming qualities of omega-3 fatty acids, this journey illuminates the importance of strategic nutrient intake. By intertwining the principles of AIP with a nuanced understanding of these nutrients, individuals with Hashimoto's can empower themselves on their path to recovery, reclaiming vitality and wellbeing one nutrient at a time.

ROLE OF SUPPLEMENTS IN AIP

The Role of Supplements in AIP for Optimal Health

The Autoimmune Protocol (AIP) diet is renowned for its emphasis on nutrient-dense, whole foods to manage autoimmune conditions and promote healing. While the foundation of AIP is centered around nourishing meals that avoid common triggers, there are instances where incorporating supplements can provide valuable support. Supplements can bridge nutritional gaps, enhance immune function, and address specific deficiencies commonly associated with autoimmune disorders. However, it's crucial to approach supplementation thoughtfully, ensuring that the chosen supplements align with the principles of AIP and your individual needs.

In this exploration of the role of supplements in the AIP journey, we'll delve into key considerations for AIP patients, discussing the supplements that hold potential benefits, their rationale, and how to integrate them effectively. From addressing common nutrient deficiencies to supporting gut health and managing inflammation, this discussion aims to offer insights into how supplements can be a complementary aspect of an AIP lifestyle. Remember, consulting with a healthcare professional or registered dietitian experienced in AIP is essential before introducing any supplements to your regimen, as personalized guidance ensures the best approach for your unique health goals.

Lifestyle and Stress Management:

Navigating the intricacies of the Autoimmune Protocol (AIP) is more than just following a dietary regimen; it's a comprehensive approach to managing autoimmune conditions and promoting overall wellness. An essential yet often overlooked aspect of this journey is the vital connection between lifestyle and stress management. Recognizing that stress can significantly impact immune function and exacerbate autoimmune symptoms, AIP patients are encouraged to embrace a holistic lifestyle that encompasses strategies to alleviate stress, nurture mental well-being, and optimize healing.

This section delves into the symbiotic relationship between lifestyle choices, stress reduction, and the success of the AIP protocol. From adopting relaxation techniques and mindful practices to fostering a supportive environment, AIP patients can empower themselves to create an atmosphere conducive to healing. By understanding how stress affects their bodies and implementing practical techniques to mitigate its effects, individuals can unlock the full potential of the AIP approach and cultivate a more balanced, health-enhancing lifestyle. In the pages that follow, we explore the transformative impact of stress management on autoimmune health, offering insights and strategies that empower AIP patients to live not only nourished, but also emotionally resilient lives.

STRESS'S IMPACT ON AUTOIMMUNITY AND HASHIMOTO'S

Navigating the intricate relationship between stress and autoimmune conditions like Hashimoto's within the framework of the Autoimmune Protocol (AIP) is a critical aspect of fostering holistic well-being. Beyond its emotional toll, stress can profoundly impact the immune system, potentially exacerbating autoimmune responses. For AIP patients, comprehending the interplay between stress and Hashimoto's is essential in their journey towards healing. Research suggests that chronic stress may contribute to inflammation, hormonal imbalances, and immune dysfunction, all of which can trigger or worsen Hashimoto's symptoms. By implementing AIP's dietary and lifestyle principles, individuals can proactively address stress, reducing its impact on autoimmune conditions. This holistic approach involves nourishing the body with nutrient-dense foods, practicing stress-relieving techniques like meditation and gentle exercise, and fostering a supportive mindset. This symbiotic relationship between AIP and stress management holds the promise of alleviating Hashimoto's symptoms and fostering a more resilient immune system.

INCORPORATING RELAXATION TECHNIQUES INTO AIP

Embarking on the Autoimmune Protocol (AIP) requires not only dietary adjustments but also a holistic approach to healing. Recognizing the intricate connection between mind and body, incorporating relaxation techniques into your AIP regimen can significantly amplify the benefits of this healing protocol. Stress, a known trigger for autoimmune responses, can impede progress. By embracing practices such as mindfulness, deep breathing, meditation, and gentle movement, AIP patients can create a harmonious environment that complements their dietary efforts. This synergy between dietary nourishment and relaxation fosters a profound sense of well-being, potentially accelerating healing and supporting a more balanced immune system. In this exploration, we delve into the transformative impact of weaving relaxation techniques into the fabric of the AIP journey, paving the way for a more empowered and holistic approach to health.

Balancing Exercise and Rest for Recovery

Embarking on the Autoimmune Protocol (AIP) is a profound step toward better health and healing. However, the road to recovery involves more than just dietary changes; it encompasses a holistic approach that includes exercise and rest. For AIP patients, finding the delicate equilibrium between physical activity and sufficient rest is crucial for supporting the body's healing processes. Engaging in appropriate exercises can boost circulation, enhance mobility, and promote overall well-being. Yet, equally important is the recognition that rest is a powerful tool in combating inflammation and allowing the body to repair. In this delicate dance between movement and stillness, understanding the types of exercises that align with AIP principles and embracing restorative practices is essential for achieving optimal recovery and long-term wellness.

Tracking and Monitoring Progress:

Embarking on the Autoimmune Protocol (AIP) journey represents a proactive step towards managing autoimmune conditions through dietary adjustments. As the AIP diet emphasizes eliminating potential triggers and fostering healing, a well-structured approach to tracking and monitoring progress becomes paramount. This practice enables individuals to gain insights into their body's response, identify patterns, and make informed decisions to optimize their wellness. In this exploration of tracking and monitoring strategies for AIP patients, we delve into the significance of personalized data collection, the tools available for effective tracking, and the holistic benefits of vigilantly observing one's progress. By cultivating this mindful awareness, AIP adherents can cultivate a deeper understanding of their body's reactions, facilitating a more tailored and impactful healing journey.

KEEPING A HASHIMOTO'S SYMPTOM JOURNAL

Navigating Hashimoto's disease while following the Autoimmune Protocol (AIP) can be a complex journey, but it's one that empowers you to take control of your health. A crucial tool in this endeavor is keeping a Hashimoto's symptom journal. This journal serves as your personalized guide, helping you track not only your dietary choices but also the intricate interplay between your symptoms, triggers, and the effectiveness of the AIP protocol. Each entry becomes a window into your body's responses, revealing patterns that might otherwise go unnoticed. From energy levels to mood swings, from digestion to inflammation, your symptom journal becomes a compass, aiding you in making informed decisions on your healing path. In this article, we'll explore the importance of maintaining a symptom journal, how to set it up effectively, and how it can work in harmony with your AIP journey to bring you closer to a life of improved well-being.

Using Biomarkers to Assess AIP's Effectiveness

For individuals navigating the Autoimmune Protocol (AIP), the journey to better health is a mindful and transformative process. As AIP's popularity grows, so does the interest in understanding its tangible effects on well-being. This is where biomarkers step in as invaluable tools. Biomarkers, measurable indicators within the body, offer a window into the effectiveness of the AIP regimen. By tracking specific markers, such as inflammation levels, immune system activity, and nutrient deficiencies, AIP patients can gain insight into how their bodies respond to dietary and lifestyle changes. This personalized approach allows for a deeper understanding of the program's impact, providing valuable data to fine-tune the AIP journey and celebrate milestones of progress. In this exploration, we delve into the significance of biomarkers in assessing the effectiveness of the AIP protocol, paving the way for informed decisions and empowered well-being.

ADAPTING AIP BASED ON INDIVIDUAL RESPONSES

The Autoimmune Protocol (AIP) stands as a powerful approach to managing autoimmune conditions through dietary choices. However, each individual's body responds uniquely to foods and lifestyle adjustments. As we embark on the journey to restore our health, it becomes evident that a one-size-fits-all approach might not fully capture our complex needs. This is where the art of adapting AIP based on individual responses comes into play. By keenly observing how our bodies react and interact with specific foods, we can tailor the AIP framework to suit our distinct requirements. This approach requires patience, mindfulness, and a willingness to explore. In this exploration, we uncover a personalized path that optimizes healing and well-being. In this guide, we delve into the nuances of individualized AIP adaptation, empowering AIP patients to forge a unique route to wellness.

Navigating Social Situations and Challenges:

Embarking on the Autoimmune Protocol (AIP) can be a transformative step towards better health, but it also brings about unique challenges when interacting in social settings. As AIP focuses on healing and managing autoimmune conditions through diet, individuals often find themselves in situations where their dietary choices stand out. From gatherings with friends and family to dining out at restaurants, maintaining AIP-compliant meals can seem daunting. Balancing the need for self-care with the desire for social engagement requires strategic planning, open communication, and a dash of creativity. In this guide, we delve into practical strategies for AIP patients to gracefully navigate social scenarios, from sharing their dietary needs with sensitivity to discovering AIP-friendly options outside their own kitchen. By empowering AIP patients with the tools to confidently handle these situations, we aim to ensure that their journey towards wellness is not only successful but also rich with positive social connections.

AIP-FRIENDLY DINING OUT AND SOCIALIZING

Navigating dining out and socializing while adhering to the Autoimmune Protocol (AIP) can be both exciting and challenging for AIP patients. While the AIP diet is designed to promote healing and reduce inflammation, it's essential to maintain the same level of diligence when enjoying meals outside the comfort of your own kitchen. AIP-friendly dining out and socializing require a blend of preparation, communication, and adaptability. From selecting the right restaurants that offer suitable options to effectively communicating your dietary needs to restaurant staff, this journey can be a rewarding one. Discovering AIP-approved menu items, understanding ingredient sourcing, and creatively modifying dishes can transform dining out into an opportunity to savor delicious flavors while staying true to your health goals. As you venture into social gatherings and restaurant experiences, arming yourself with knowledge and strategies will empower you to relish the pleasures of food and company without compromising your AIP commitment.

Dealing with AIP Challenges in Everyday Life

Dealing with AIP challenges in everyday life requires not only dedication but also a thoughtful approach to overcome obstacles and maintain a fulfilling lifestyle. From reshaping long-standing habits to making informed choices at every meal, the path to healing can sometimes be daunting. This guide delves into the practical aspects of embracing AIP principles while gracefully addressing the common hurdles that arise. We'll explore strategies for dining out, managing social situations, and finding convenience in a world saturated with processed foods. Additionally, we'll tackle the emotional aspects of adjusting to a new way of eating, offering insights into maintaining a positive mindset and seeking support. By acknowledging the intricacies of the AIP journey and equipping ourselves with effective coping mechanisms, we empower AIP patients to not only navigate challenges but also thrive in their pursuit of improved health and well-being.

2

UTILIZING THE AIP

The Autoimmune Protocol (AIP) has emerged as a promising approach for individuals seeking to recover from Hashimoto's Thyroiditis, an autoimmune disorder that affects the thyroid gland. Hashimoto's is characterized by the immune system mistakenly attacking the thyroid tissue, leading to inflammation and a range of symptoms such as fatigue, weight gain, and mood disturbances. AIP offers a comprehensive dietary and lifestyle strategy aimed at reducing inflammation, restoring gut health, and promoting overall well-being. Let's delve into how individuals can effectively utilize the AIP to aid in their journey toward Hashimoto's recovery.

At the core of the AIP lies a strategic dietary plan that emphasizes the elimination of certain foods known to trigger inflammation and immune responses. The Elimination Phase of the AIP involves cutting out potentially problematic foods such as grains, legumes, dairy, processed sugars, and nightshade vegetables. By removing these potential triggers, the immune system's hyperactivity is mitigated, giving the body a chance to heal.

AIP-friendly foods are those that provide essential nutrients while minimizing inflammation. Nutrient-dense choices like lean meats, fish, non-starchy vegetables, and healthy fats form the foundation of the AIP diet. These foods are rich in vitamins, minerals, and antioxidants, which play a vital role in reducing oxidative stress and supporting the immune system. By emphasizing nutrient density, individuals can nourish their bodies while promoting healing.

Inflammation and gut health are intricately linked, and addressing gut issues is a cornerstone of the AIP approach. Leaky gut, a condition where the intestinal barrier becomes compromised, can exacerbate autoimmune responses. The AIP diet's exclusion of potential irritants gives the gut a chance to repair and regenerate. Additionally, the AIP promotes the consumption of gut-friendly foods like bone broth and fermented foods that aid in gut restoration.

Managing Hashimoto's symptoms requires more than just dietary adjustments. AIP recognizes the importance of stress management and lifestyle modifications in the recovery process. Stress has been shown to exacerbate autoimmune conditions, including Hashimoto's. Incorporating relaxation techniques like meditation, yoga, and mindfulness can help regulate the stress response and promote hormonal balance.

Meal planning is essential to successful AIP implementation. Crafting balanced meals that adhere to the protocol can initially be challenging, but resources such as AIP-friendly recipes, cookbooks, and online communities provide valuable guidance. Batch cooking and meal prepping can simplify the process, ensuring that compliant meals are readily available.

Tracking progress is another crucial aspect of utilizing the AIP effectively. Keeping a symptom journal can help individuals identify patterns, pinpoint trigger foods, and monitor improvements over time. Regular consultations with healthcare professionals are essential for interpreting these changes and making necessary adjustments to the AIP plan.

Social situations and challenges can present hurdles in AIP adherence. Dining out or attending social gatherings can be daunting, but with proper preparation, it's possible to maintain the protocol while still participating in these activities.

Communicating dietary needs with hosts or restaurants and bringing AIP-friendly options can help individuals navigate these scenarios.

While the Elimination Phase is vital for calming the immune system and promoting healing, it's not meant to be followed indefinitely. Reintroducing eliminated foods systematically and under the guidance of a healthcare professional allows individuals to identify which foods may trigger reactions, and which can be safely incorporated back into their diet.

The Autoimmune Protocol (AIP) presents a comprehensive and holistic approach for individuals recovering from Hashimoto's Thyroiditis. By utilizing the AIP's principles of dietary modification, gut health restoration, stress management, and lifestyle adjustments, individuals can embark on a path to recovery that not only addresses their symptoms but also supports their overall well-being. However, it's important to note that AIP is not a one-size-fits-all solution, and personalized guidance from healthcare professionals is essential for tailoring the approach to individual needs and circumstances.

3

BREAKFASTS

AIP (Autoimmune Protocol) breakfasts are an essential part of the dietary approach for individuals seeking to manage autoimmune conditions, such as Hashimoto's Thyroiditis. These breakfast options focus on nutrient-dense, anti-inflammatory foods while avoiding common triggers that could exacerbate symptoms. Here are some delicious and nourishing AIP breakfast ideas to kick-start your day:

1.Sweet Potato Hash: Sautéed sweet potatoes with cooked ground turkey or pork, sautéed spinach, and diced apples. Season with AIP-approved herbs and spices like garlic, thyme, and rosemary.

2.Coconut-Crusted Chicken Tenders: Dip chicken tenders in coconut flour, then coconut milk, and finally, shredded coconut. Bake until crispy and serve with a side of fresh fruit or AIP-friendly dipping sauce.

3.Turmeric Cauliflower Rice Bowl: Sauté cauliflower rice with turmeric, ground beef or turkey, and a variety of chopped vegetables like carrots, zucchini, and bell peppers. Top with fresh herbs and a drizzle of olive oil.

4. Baked Avocado Eggs: Slice an avocado in half and remove the pit. Scoop out a bit of flesh to make room for an egg. Crack an egg into each avocado half and bake until the egg is cooked to your liking.

5. Berry Coconut Smoothie: Blend coconut milk, mixed berries (blueberries, strawberries, raspberries), and a scoop of collagen powder. Add a handful of greens like spinach or kale for an extra nutritional boost.

6. Plantain Pancakes: Mash ripe plantains and mix with coconut flour, a pinch of baking soda, and a dash of cinnamon. Cook spoonfuls of batter on a skillet with coconut oil until golden brown.

7. Breakfast Sausage Patties: Make your own AIP-friendly sausage patties using ground pork or turkey and AIP-approved herbs and spices like sage, thyme, and oregano.

8. Zucchini Noodles with Pesto: Spiralize zucchini into noodles and toss with homemade basil and avocado pesto. Add cooked and shredded chicken for extra protein.

9. AIP-friendly Porridge: Combine mashed cooked sweet potatoes or plantains with coconut milk, cinnamon, and a touch of maple syrup (if tolerated). Top with toasted coconut flakes and chopped nuts (if allowed).

10. Smoked Salmon Wraps: Wrap smoked salmon around cucumber slices, jicama sticks, or avocado slices. Drizzle with lemon juice and sprinkle with fresh dill.

11. Savory Breakfast Bowl: Sauté ground turkey or beef with kale, chopped carrots, and butternut squash. Season with AIP-approved spices and top with sliced green onions.

12. Baked Apple with Cinnamon: Core an apple and fill the center with coconut oil, cinnamon, and a sprinkle of raisins. Bake until the apple is tender.

4

VEGETABLES

Good vegetables play a crucial role in the diet of individuals following the Autoimmune Protocol (AIP), as they provide essential nutrients and contribute to overall health and wellness. AIP is a dietary approach designed to help manage autoimmune conditions by focusing on nutrient-dense, anti-inflammatory foods. Here are some excellent vegetables that can be included in an AIP patient's diet

1. Leafy Greens (e.g., kale, spinach, collard greens): These vibrant greens are rich in vitamins A, C, and K, as well as minerals like iron and calcium. They are known for their anti-inflammatory properties and can help support the immune system. Leafy greens can be used as a base for salads or added to soups and stews.

2. Sweet Potatoes: Sweet potatoes are a nutrient powerhouse, packed with vitamin A, vitamin C, and dietary fiber. They have a naturally sweet flavor and can be roasted, mashed, or turned into fries. Their complex carbohydrates provide sustained energy and can help stabilize blood sugar levels.

3. Zucchini: Zucchini is a versatile vegetable that can be spiralized into noodles or sliced and added to stir-fries. It is low in carbohydrates and calories while providing vitamins B6 and C. Zucchini is also a good source of dietary fiber, aiding in digestion and gut health.

4. Carrots: Carrots are known for their high beta-carotene content, which is converted to vitamin A in the body. Vitamin A is essential for maintaining healthy skin, vision, and immune function. Carrots can be enjoyed raw as a crunchy snack or cooked in various dishes.

5. Cauliflower: Cauliflower is a versatile vegetable that can be used as a low-carb substitute for rice or mashed potatoes. It's a good source of vitamin C, fiber, and antioxidants. Cauliflower contains compounds that support detoxification and reduce inflammation.

6. Beets: Beets are rich in antioxidants and nitrates, which can help improve blood flow and cardiovascular health. They can be roasted, boiled, or grated raw into salads. Beets' vibrant color is a sign of their high nutrient content.

7. Broccoli: Broccoli is a cruciferous vegetable that contains sulforaphane, a compound known for its

anti-inflammatory and antioxidant properties. It's also a great source of vitamin K, vitamin C, and fiber. Broccoli can be steamed, roasted, or added to casseroles.

8. Cabbage: Cabbage is another cruciferous vegetable that supports gut health due to its fiber content and potential probiotic properties. It's also rich in vitamins K and C. Cabbage can be used to make slaws, sauerkraut, or added to soups.

9. Parsnips: Parsnips are a root vegetable that offers a slightly sweet flavor. They contain dietary fiber, vitamin C, and folate. Roasting parsnips can enhance their natural sweetness and provide a satisfying side dish.

10. Swiss Chard: Swiss chard is a colorful leafy green that provides vitamins A, C, and K. It also contains magnesium, which is important for muscle and nerve function. Swiss chard can be sautéed or added to omelets for a nutrient boost.

Incorporating these vegetables into an AIP patient's diet can provide a wide range of nutrients while supporting their immune system and overall health. It's important to choose organic, fresh, and locally sourced produce whenever possible to maximize the benefits of these nutrient-rich vegetables. Always consult with a healthcare professional or registered dietitian before making significant dietary changes, especially for individuals with specific health conditions like autoimmune disorders.

5

POULTRY DISHES

Delicious Poultry Dishes for AIP Patients: Nourishment and Flavor in Harmony

For individuals following the Autoimmune Protocol (AIP), a diet designed to alleviate symptoms of autoimmune disorders, finding suitable and appetizing meal options is crucial. Poultry dishes offer a wide range of flavorful and nutrient-dense choices that align well with the AIP guidelines. Here, we explore some delectable poultry dishes along with their descriptions and the benefits they provide to AIP patients.

1. Herb-Roasted Chicken with Root Vegetables:

A succulent herb-roasted chicken, accompanied by an array of colorful root vegetables such as sweet potatoes, carrots, and parsnips, forms a hearty and wholesome meal. The chicken is seasoned with AIP-friendly herbs like thyme, rosemary, and oregano, which not only enhance the flavor but also provide anti-inflammatory and antioxidant benefits. Root vegetables offer dietary fiber, vitamins, and minerals, aiding in gut health and immune system support.

2. Lemon-Herb Grilled Turkey Breast

Lean turkey breast marinated in a zesty blend of lemon juice, garlic, and AIP-compliant herbs is a lean protein option bursting with flavor. Turkey is rich in amino acids and minerals like zinc, which is essential for immune function. The zingy lemon marinade adds a refreshing twist while contributing to digestion and alkalizing the body.

3. Coconut-Curry Chicken Stew:

A fragrant coconut-curry chicken stew combines the creaminess of coconut milk with the warmth of aromatic spices. This dish can be loaded with vegetables like bell peppers, spinach, and zucchini. The coconut milk provides healthy fats while the spices, such as turmeric and ginger, possess potent anti-inflammatory properties that align perfectly with the AIP guidelines.

4. Garlic-Herb Roasted Quail:

Quail, a smaller yet flavorful poultry option, can be seasoned with garlic, thyme, and AIP-approved seasonings before being roasted to perfection. Quail is a great source of protein and B vitamins, essential for energy production and immune health. The garlic and herbs contribute to cardiovascular health and immune system modulation.

5. Rosemary Roasted Duck with Balsamic-Glazed Brussels Sprouts:

Indulge in the richness of duck meat seasoned with rosemary and roasted until crispy. Alongside, balsamic-glazed Brussels sprouts offer a delightful balance of sweetness and tanginess. Duck meat is an excellent source of iron and selenium, aiding in red blood cell formation and thyroid function. The Brussels sprouts provide fiber and antioxidants that support digestion and overall well-being.

Benefits for AIP Patients:

These poultry dishes offer numerous benefits tailored to the needs of AIP patients:

1. Lean Protein: Poultry is a fantastic source of lean protein, which is vital for tissue repair and immune system strength. AIP patients require adequate protein intake to support healing and recovery.

2. Anti-Inflammatory Properties: The herbs and spices used in these dishes, such as turmeric, ginger, and rosemary, possess anti-inflammatory properties that can help manage autoimmune symptoms.

3. Nutrient Density: Poultry dishes are rich in essential nutrients like zinc, iron, B vitamins, and healthy fats, which are crucial for immune function, energy production, and overall well-being.

4. Gut Health: The inclusion of colorful vegetables and root vegetables in these dishes promotes a diverse gut microbiome, supporting digestion and immune system balance.

5. Variety and Flavor: AIP patients often face dietary restrictions, making variety important. These dishes offer a range of flavors and ingredients, making the AIP journey more enjoyable.

Incorporating these poultry dishes into an AIP meal plan can provide nourishment, flavor, and therapeutic benefits. However, individual tolerances may vary, so it's important for AIP patients to consult with a healthcare professional or registered dietitian before making significant changes to their diet. With creativity in the kitchen and a focus on nutrient-rich ingredients, AIP patients can savor both healing and deliciousness in each bite.

6

SEAFOOD

The Autoimmune Protocol (AIP) diet is gaining recognition for its potential to alleviate autoimmune conditions by reducing inflammation and promoting gut health. Seafood, rich in omega-3 fatty acids and other essential nutrients, can play a crucial role in an AIP patient's diet. This article explores a variety of delectable seafood options, providing both enticing descriptions and insights into their benefits for individuals following the AIP protocol.

Salmon: The Omega-3 Powerhouse

Salmon, with its succulent flesh and rich flavor, is a top choice for AIP patients seeking both taste and health benefits. This fatty fish is renowned for its high omega-3 fatty acid content, specifically EPA and DHA, which are known to reduce inflammation and support cardiovascular health. Additionally, salmon provides essential protein and a range of vitamins and minerals that are vital for overall well-being. Whether grilled, baked, or broiled, salmon's versatility ensures it's a palate-pleasing delight for AIP-compliant meals.

Sardines: Tiny Fish, Mighty Nutrients

Sardines may be small, but they are a nutritional powerhouse, making them an excellent choice for those on the AIP diet. Packed with omega-3s, calcium, vitamin D, and coenzyme Q10, sardines contribute to bone health, cardiovascular support, and improved energy production. Their intense flavor lends itself well to salads, spreads, or simply enjoyed straight from the can, providing AIP patients with a convenient and nourishing seafood option.

Mackerel: Flavorful and Satisfying

Mackerel's bold, robust flavor makes it a favorite among seafood enthusiasts. For AIP patients, mackerel offers more than just taste – it's a rich source of omega-3s, selenium, and vitamin B12. These nutrients aid in reducing inflammation, supporting thyroid function, and promoting healthy nervous system function. Mackerel's distinctive taste stands up well to grilling or pan-searing, making it an appetizing choice for AIP-compliant dishes.

Cod: Mild Delicacy with Abundant Benefits

Known for its mild flavor and delicate texture, cod is a versatile seafood option that pairs well with various AIP-friendly ingredients. Cod is a reliable source of lean protein, phosphorus, and vitamin B12, which aids in energy production and nerve health. Moreover, its low mercury content makes it a safe choice for regular consumption. Whether baked, poached, or pan-fried, cod's subtle taste makes it a canvas for creative AIP recipes.

Scallops: Tender Indulgence with Nutrient Bounty

Scallops offer AIP patients a luxurious seafood experience with their tender, melt-in-your-mouth texture. These shellfish are rich in vitamin B12, magnesium, and zinc – essential nutrients for immune function, energy metabolism, and skin health. Scallops' delicate taste pairs well with AIP-compliant sauces and garnishes, allowing for elegant and nourishing dishes that support autoimmune healing.

Shrimp: Versatile and Nutrient-Rich

Shrimp's widespread popularity is attributed to its versatility and delightful taste. For AIP patients, shrimp provides a good source of protein, iodine, and selenium. Iodine is essential for thyroid function, while selenium supports the immune system and antioxidant defenses. Whether grilled, sautéed, or incorporated into soups, shrimp's adaptable nature ensures a variety of delectable options within the AIP framework.

Benefits for AIP Patients

1. Anti-Inflammatory Properties: Omega-3 fatty acids found in seafood play a pivotal role in reducing inflammation, a key factor in autoimmune conditions. Incorporating seafood into the AIP diet can help manage inflammation and alleviate symptoms.

2. Nutrient Density: Seafood offers a plethora of essential nutrients such as omega-3s, vitamins, minerals, and antioxidants. These nutrients support overall health, aid in tissue repair, and contribute to optimal immune function.

3. Gut Health: A healthy gut is vital for autoimmune management. Seafood's nutrient profile includes compounds that support gut lining integrity and promote a balanced gut microbiome.

4. Heart Health: Omega-3s in seafood are renowned for their cardiovascular benefits, including improved cholesterol levels, reduced blood pressure, and enhanced heart function – all crucial aspects for individuals with autoimmune concerns.

5. Skin and Joint Health: The nutrients present in seafood can contribute to healthier skin and joint function, areas often affected by autoimmune conditions.

Incorporating a variety of seafood into the Autoimmune Protocol (AIP) diet can offer individuals not only delectable flavors but also a host of health benefits. From the omega-3-rich salmon to the nutrient-packed sardines, each seafood choice provides unique advantages for AIP patients seeking to manage their autoimmune conditions. By embracing these flavorful options, AIP patients can savor the tastes of the sea while nurturing their bodies on the path to healing.

7

BEEF AND PORK

For individuals adhering to the Autoimmune Protocol (AIP) diet, selecting the right sources of protein is crucial to support their healing journey. Beef and pork, two protein-packed meats, offer a plethora of nutrients that can play a pivotal role in the well-being of AIP patients. With their rich taste and diverse culinary potential, beef and pork are not only satisfying but also provide essential nutrients necessary for healing and maintaining optimal health.

The Nutrient Profile of Beef

Beef, derived from cattle, is renowned for its robust flavor and tender texture. Grass-fed and pasture-raised beef is particularly favored within the AIP community due to its superior nutrient composition. Rich in high-quality protein, beef is an excellent source of essential amino acids that are vital for repairing tissues and supporting immune function. Beef is also abundant in vitamins and minerals, including B-vitamins like B12 and B6, zinc, iron, and selenium.

Zinc, found abundantly in beef, is critical for immune system regulation and cellular repair. For AIP patients dealing with autoimmune disorders, zinc plays a pivotal role in modulating immune responses and maintaining skin health. Iron, another essential mineral present in beef, supports oxygen transport within the body, making it particularly beneficial for individuals dealing with fatigue often associated with autoimmune conditions.

The Nutrient Profile of Pork

Pork, derived from pigs, offers a diverse array of cuts, each with its own flavor profile and culinary possibilities. Like beef, the nutritional value of pork is enhanced when sourced from animals raised in free-range or pasture-based systems. Pork is a versatile protein source that provides essential amino acids, making it an ideal component of an AIP-friendly diet.

Pork is an excellent source of B-vitamins such as thiamin (B1), riboflavin (B2), and niacin (B3), which are essential for energy production, nerve function, and overall metabolic health. Additionally, pork contains phosphorus, a mineral that contributes to bone health and cell repair. AIP patients often seek phosphorus-rich foods to support tissue healing, making pork an appealing choice.

Benefits for AIP Patients

1. High-Quality Protein: Both beef and pork offer complete proteins, supplying the body with the essential amino acids required for tissue repair and immune function. This is crucial for AIP patients whose immune systems may be compromised due to autoimmune conditions.

2. Vitamins and Minerals: Beef and pork are rich sources of various vitamins and minerals that support overall health. B-vitamins are essential for energy production and nervous system health, which are vital for AIP patients aiming to regain their energy levels and support their nervous system.

3. Zinc for Immune Support: The high zinc content in beef aids in immune system regulation, assisting AIP patients in managing autoimmune responses. Zinc also supports wound healing and skin health, addressing common challenges faced by individuals with autoimmune disorders.

4. Iron for Energy and Healing: The iron content in both beef and pork is beneficial for AIP patients

dealing with fatigue and anemia. Adequate iron intake supports oxygen transport and tissue healing, helping patients regain their vitality.

5. Phosphorus for Tissue Repair: Pork's phosphorus content aids in tissue repair and maintenance, which is essential for AIP patients working towards healing their bodies from the inside out.

6. Diverse Culinary Options: Both beef and pork offer a wide variety of cuts that can be prepared in numerous ways, catering to the preferences and dietary restrictions of AIP patients. This culinary versatility prevents monotony in their diet and encourages adherence to the AIP protocol.

Bringing in nutrient-dense beef and pork into an AIP-friendly diet can provide numerous benefits to individuals navigating autoimmune conditions. From their protein content and array of vitamins and minerals to their immune-supporting properties, these meats offer a well-rounded package of nutrients that align with the healing goals of AIP patients. However, it's essential to prioritize grass-fed, pasture-raised, and high-quality sources of beef and pork to maximize their health benefits and ensure they align with the principles of the Autoimmune Protocol. As always, consulting a healthcare professional or nutritionist is advisable before making significant dietary changes, especially for those with specific health concerns.

8

SNACKS AND SWEET TREATS

Delicious and Nourishing Snacks and Sweet Treats for AIP Patients

For individuals following the Autoimmune Protocol (AIP) diet, finding satisfying and flavorful snacks and sweet treats can be a rewarding endeavor. The AIP diet is designed to mitigate inflammation and promote healing by eliminating potentially trigger-inducing foods. While adhering to these dietary restrictions, it's essential to discover snacks and treats that not only comply with the protocol but also delight the taste buds and provide essential nutrients.

Snack Sensations:

1. Crispy Kale Chips: These crispy, oven-baked kale chips offer a satisfying crunch and are rich in vitamins and minerals. Drizzled with olive oil and sprinkled with AIP-approved seasonings like sea salt or nutritional yeast, they're a delicious and nutrient-packed snack.

2. Avocado Boats: Sliced avocado halves filled with diced mango, shredded coconut, and a drizzle of

lemon juice make for a refreshing and nourishing snack. Avocado provides healthy fats and vitamins, while mango adds natural sweetness.

3. Cucumber and Guacamole Bites:** Thin cucumber slices topped with guacamole create a cool and creamy snack. Avocado, a staple in AIP diets, supplies monounsaturated fats that support heart health and reduce inflammation.

Sweet Delights:

1. Baked Apples with Cinnamon: Baking apple slices sprinkled with cinnamon results in a warm and comforting treat. Apples offer dietary fiber and antioxidants, while cinnamon adds a burst of flavor without compromising AIP guidelines.

2. Coconut Berry Parfait: Layers of coconut yogurt and mixed berries create a visually appealing and indulgent treat. Coconut yogurt is a dairy-free alternative that aligns with the AIP diet, and berries provide essential vitamins and antioxidants.

3. Tigernut Energy Balls: Tigernuts, a nut-free tuber, can be transformed into energy balls with dates, coconut, and a touch of vanilla. These bite-sized treats offer natural sweetness and a dose of fiber, aiding digestion.

The Benefits:

1. Nutrient Density: AIP-friendly snacks and sweet treats often incorporate nutrient-dense ingredients like avocados, berries, kale, and tigernuts. These foods are rich in vitamins, minerals, and antioxidants that support overall health and aid in the healing process.

2. Balanced Blood Sugar: Many AIP-compliant snacks and treats are naturally low in added sugars and refined carbohydrates, helping to stabilize blood sugar levels. This is especially important for individuals with autoimmune conditions, as blood sugar imbalances can contribute to inflammation.

3. Inflammation Management: The AIP diet aims to reduce inflammation, and the selected snacks and treats align with this goal. The ingredients used are carefully chosen to avoid common triggers and promote healing, making them suitable choices for AIP patients.

4. Variety and Enjoyment: Following a restricted diet can sometimes lead to monotony. Incorporating diverse and flavorful snacks and treats keeps the AIP journey enjoyable and prevents feelings of deprivation.

AIP patients can savor a range of delectable snacks and sweet treats that align with their dietary requirements and health objectives. From nutrient-packed kale chips to luscious coconut berry parfaits, these options cater to taste preferences while providing essential nutrients, supporting inflammation management, and contributing to overall well-being.

9

SAUCES, STAPLES

Sauces play a pivotal role in transforming simple dishes into culinary delights, enhancing taste and texture while providing a myriad of benefits for those following the Autoimmune Protocol (AIP) diet. AIP focuses on eliminating potential trigger foods to mitigate inflammation and promote healing. While navigating this dietary journey might seem challenging, the incorporation of AIP-friendly sauces can greatly diversify meals, making them both flavorful and nourishing.

1. Coconut Aminos: This versatile sauce stands as a brilliant alternative to soy sauce, a common AIP exclusion due to its inflammatory properties. Derived from coconut sap, coconut aminos offer a slightly sweet and savory flavor, perfect for seasoning meats, vegetables, and stir-fries. Rich in amino acids, vitamins, and minerals, this sauce supports immune function and aids in tissue repair.

2. Avocado Pesto: Made with fresh basil, avocado, olive oil, and garlic, this sauce caters to AIP requirements while delivering a burst of vibrant flavors. Avocado's healthy fats and anti-

inflammatory compounds pair well with nutrient-dense basil, creating a sauce that can elevate zucchini noodles, roasted chicken, or as a dip for veggie sticks.

3. Bone Broth Gravy: AIP encourages the consumption of nutrient-rich bone broth, and crafting a gravy from it adds depth to dishes while nurturing the gut lining. Combining bone broth with arrowroot starch or coconut flour results in a luscious gravy that complements roasted meats, mashed sweet potatoes, and cauliflower.

4. Turmeric Tahini Dressing: Tahini, made from sesame seeds, forms the base of this dressing, which is enriched with anti-inflammatory turmeric and a hint of lemon juice. Drizzle it over salads or use it as a dip for roasted vegetables to infuse your meals with wholesome fats and healing properties.

5. Apple-Cinnamon BBQ Sauce: Ditching the conventional sugar-laden BBQ sauce, this AIP-friendly version employs applesauce and aromatic spices to create a delightful condiment. The blend of sweet and savory flavors brings out the best in grilled meats, adding antioxidants and natural sweetness without causing inflammation.

6. Ginger-Lime Dressing: A fusion of zesty lime and soothing ginger creates a dressing that adds a refreshing twist to salads and grilled seafood. Ginger's anti-inflammatory compounds support digestive health, making this sauce a valuable addition to an AIP-friendly regimen.

7. Roasted Garlic and Lemon Aioli: Crafting a dairy-free aioli using roasted garlic, lemon juice, and olive oil results in a rich, creamy sauce that pairs well with grilled meats, roasted vegetables, and even AIP-friendly cassava fries. Roasted garlic offers prebiotic benefits for gut health, while lemon adds a burst of vitamin C.

Incorporating these sauces into the AIP diet offers not only a vast array of flavors but also significant health benefits. AIP patients can relish their meals without compromising their healing journey. These sauces align with AIP principles, devoid of common allergens and inflammation triggers, making them perfect allies for those seeking to manage autoimmune conditions through dietary means. From nourishing bone broth gravies to invigorating ginger-lime dressings, these sauces turn AIP meals into delightful feasts, contributing to both flavor satisfaction and overall wellness.

10

MEAL PLANNING

Becoming an AIP (Autoimmune Protocol) pro meal planner requires a combination of careful preparation, creativity, and a deep understanding of AIP-compliant foods. By mastering the art of AIP meal planning, you can effectively manage your autoimmune condition while enjoying flavorful and nourishing meals. Here's how to become an AIP pro meal planner:

1. EDUCATE YOURSELF: Start by thoroughly familiarizing yourself with the principles of the AIP. Understand which foods are allowed and which ones should be avoided during the elimination phase. Research nutrient-dense options to ensure you're getting a variety of vitamins and minerals.

Educating yourself on using the Autoimmune Protocol (AIP) to treat Hashimoto's Thyroiditis is a crucial step towards effectively managing this autoimmune condition and promoting your overall well-being. Hashimoto's Thyroiditis is characterized by an immune system attack on the thyroid gland, leading to inflammation, hormonal imbalances, and a range of symptoms. AIP is a comprehensive approach that focuses on dietary and lifestyle modifications to reduce inflammation, support the immune system, and potentially alleviate symptoms. Here's how to educate yourself on using AIP to treat Hashimoto's:

Understand Hashimoto's Thyroiditis: Begin by familiarizing yourself with the basics of Hashimoto's. Learn about the autoimmune nature of the condition, its impact on thyroid function, and the potential symptoms that can arise.

Research AIP Principles: Dive into the foundational principles of the Autoimmune Protocol. Understand why certain foods are eliminated during the initial phase, the rationale behind nutrient-dense choices, and how AIP aims to restore gut health and immune balance.

Explore AIP-Friendly Foods: Learn about the foods that are encouraged and those that are restricted on the AIP. Discover nutrient-rich options like lean meats, fish, vegetables, fruits, and healthy fats that can support your body's healing process.

Study Inflammation and Gut Health: Delve into the connection between inflammation, gut health, and autoimmune conditions. Understand how leaky gut syndrome can contribute to Hashimoto's and how the AIP's emphasis on gut restoration can benefit your overall health.

Consult Reliable Resources: Turn to reputable sources such as books, articles, and websites written by healthcare professionals, nutritionists, and individuals who have successfully used AIP to manage Hashimoto's. Look for evidence-based information and personal experiences.

Seek Professional Guidance: Consider working with a healthcare practitioner who is knowledgeable about Hashimoto's and the AIP. They can provide personalized advice, help you create a tailored AIP plan, and monitor your progress.

Join Supportive Communities: Engage with online forums, social media groups, and local meetups focused on AIP and autoimmune health. Connecting with others who are on a similar journey can provide valuable insights, encouragement, and a sense of community.

Experiment with Recipes: Explore AIP-friendly recipes and meal plans that cater to Hashimoto's management. Experiment with different ingredients, flavors, and cooking techniques to keep your meals enjoyable and satisfying.

Track Your Progress: Keep a journal to document your symptoms, dietary changes, and how you feel throughout your AIP journey. This can help you identify patterns, trigger foods, and improvements in your health.

Stay Open-Minded: Recognize that the AIP may require adjustments and individualization. Listen to your body, be patient with the process, and be willing to adapt your approach based on your unique needs and responses.

Educating yourself about using AIP to treat Hashimoto's Thyroiditis empowers you to take an active role in your health. By becoming well-informed, you can make informed decisions, confidently navigate the AIP journey, and work towards managing your Hashimoto's symptoms and achieving a better quality of life. Remember, it's always advisable to consult with a healthcare professional before making significant dietary or lifestyle changes, especially when managing a medical condition.

2. STOCK YOUR KITCHEN: Keep your kitchen well-stocked with AIP-friendly staples such as lean meats, seafood, vegetables, fruits, coconut products, and approved cooking fats. This ensures

you have the necessary ingredients on hand to create balanced meals.

Stocking your kitchen for the Autoimmune Protocol (AIP) is a pivotal step in successfully adopting this healing dietary approach. Focus on AIP-compliant staples like lean meats, seafood, a variety of fresh vegetables, and low-sugar fruits. Include nutrient-dense options such as organ meats, bone broth, and coconut products. Opt for cooking fats like coconut oil, olive oil, and avocado oil. Keep your pantry well-supplied with AIP-friendly herbs, spices, and seasonings to enhance flavor. Steer clear of grains, legumes, dairy, processed foods, and nightshades. Prioritize high-quality, sustainable ingredients to ensure your meals are both nourishing and supportive of your immune system. By thoughtfully stocking your kitchen with AIP-approved foods, you'll set yourself up for success, making meal preparation and adherence to the protocol more manageable and effective in addressing autoimmune concerns like Hashimoto's.

3. PLAN AHEAD: Set aside dedicated time each week for meal planning. Choose recipes that align with AIP guidelines and suit your preferences. Consider batch cooking, which allows you to

prepare larger quantities of food that can be easily reheated throughout the week.

Planning ahead is key when adopting the Autoimmune Protocol (AIP). Prepare by researching AIP-friendly recipes, creating a weekly meal plan, and compiling a detailed grocery list. Batch cooking proteins, chopping vegetables, and prepping snacks can save time during busy days. Plan for work or outings by packing AIP-compliant meals or snacks to avoid temptation. Having AIP-approved sauces, dressings, and condiments on hand enhances flavor and variety. Embrace flexibility, knowing that occasional adjustments may be needed. Planning ahead not only simplifies mealtime decisions but also ensures that you consistently nourish your body with nutrient-dense foods while successfully adhering to the AIP, promoting your well-being and managing autoimmune conditions like Hashimoto's Thyroiditis effectively.

4. CREATE BALANCED MEALS: Aim for balanced meals that include protein, healthy fats, and a variety of colorful vegetables. Incorporate nutrient-rich options like organ meats, bone broth, and fermented foods to support gut health.

Creating balanced meals on the Autoimmune Protocol (AIP) is key to supporting your health while managing conditions like Hashimoto's Thyroiditis. Aim to incorporate a variety of nutrient-dense foods that promote healing and reduce inflammation. Start with a foundation of high-quality protein sources such as grass-fed meats, wild-caught fish, and poultry. These provide essential amino acids for tissue repair and immune function.

Next, fill your plate with an array of colorful non-starchy vegetables like leafy greens, broccoli, and cauliflower. These veggies offer vitamins, minerals, and antioxidants that contribute to overall well-being. Include healthy fats like avocados, coconut oil, and olive oil to provide energy and aid in nutrient absorption.

To enhance gut health, consider including fermented foods like sauerkraut or kombucha. These support a balanced gut microbiome, which plays a crucial role in immune regulation.

Remember to moderate fruit consumption, opting for low-sugar options like berries that won't spike blood sugar levels. Experiment with AIP-approved herbs, spices, and seasonings to add flavor and depth to your meals.

Creating balanced AIP meals involves thoughtful planning and mindful combination of macronutrients. Prioritize nutrient density, variety, and portion control to ensure your meals are both satisfying and supportive of your healing journey. Consulting a healthcare professional or registered dietitian can provide personalized guidance as you design balanced meals tailored to your unique needs and preferences.

5. EMBRACE VARIETY: Explore different cooking methods, herbs, and spices to add variety to your meals. Experiment with unique combinations of flavors and textures to keep your palate engaged.

Embracing variety within the Autoimmune Protocol (AIP) is not only a delightful culinary adventure but also a strategic approach to optimizing health while managing conditions like Hashimoto's Thyroiditis. AIP encourages the exploration of a diverse range of nutrient-rich foods to provide essential vitamins, minerals, and antioxidants. Rotate protein sources such as grass-fed meats, wild-caught fish, and poultry to ensure a balanced amino acid profile. Incorporate a spectrum of colorful vegetables and low-sugar fruits to maximize phytonutrient intake. Experiment with alternative starches like sweet potatoes, cassava, and plantains to diversify carbohydrate sources.

Herbs and spices play a crucial role in AIP, offering both flavor and potential health benefits. Ginger, turmeric, garlic, and fresh herbs infuse dishes with anti-inflammatory and antioxidant properties. Be open to trying new cooking techniques, from roasting and steaming to fermenting and slow cooking, to enhance textures and flavors.

By embracing culinary variety, you prevent monotony, reduce the risk of nutrient deficiencies, and promote gut health through exposure to different fibers. Remember, AIP is a personalized journey, so observe how your body responds to different foods and combinations to tailor your approach. A vibrant and varied AIP menu can make the healing process enjoyable and sustainable while supporting your path to better well-being.

6. PREP INGREDIENTS: Wash, chop, and portion out ingredients in advance to streamline cooking. Prepping vegetables, marinating proteins, and having grab-and-go snacks prepared can save time during busy weekdays.

Preparing ingredients for the Autoimmune Protocol (AIP) is a strategic approach that streamlines your meal preparation, making it easier to adhere to the dietary guidelines and support your health goals. Begin by washing, chopping, and portioning out vegetables, fruits, and protein sources in advance. This step saves time and effort during busy days, allowing you to quickly assemble balanced AIP-friendly meals.

Marinating proteins ahead of time enhances flavor and reduces cooking time. Utilize AIP-approved marinades featuring herbs, citrus, and compliant oils. Batch cook proteins like chicken, beef, or fish and store them for later use. Additionally, consider roasting or sautéing a variety of vegetables and keeping them refrigerated to add to salads, stir-fries, or as side dishes throughout the week.

Preparing AIP-compliant snacks, such as sliced vegetables with guacamole or homemade fruit and coconut milk gelatin cups, ensures you have convenient and satisfying options readily available.

By prepping ingredients in advance, you're more likely to stay on track with your AIP journey. Not only does it simplify the cooking process, but it also reduces decision fatigue, making it easier to make health-conscious choices and maintain your commitment to managing autoimmune conditions like Hashimoto's Thyroiditis.

7. USE MEAL TEMPLATES: Develop meal templates that make planning easier. For example, a template could include a protein source, a selection of vegetables, and a healthy fat. Swap out components while sticking to AIP guidelines.

Using meal templates for the Autoimmune Protocol (AIP) can simplify the process of planning and preparing AIP-compliant meals while ensuring variety and nutritional balance. A meal template serves as a flexible guide, helping you create well-rounded dishes within the constraints of the protocol.

Start with a base of AIP-friendly protein sources, such as lean meats, poultry, fish, or organ meats. Pair the protein with a diverse array of non-starchy vegetables, incorporating different colors and textures to maximize nutrient intake. These veggies can be sautéed, roasted, or enjoyed raw.

Include a source of healthy fats, like avocado, coconut, or olive oil, which not only enhance flavor but also provide satiety and support immune function. Fresh herbs, garlic, ginger, and AIP-approved spices can elevate taste while offering potential health benefits.

For added nourishment, consider including bone broth or collagen-rich foods to promote gut health and support connective tissues. Additionally, incorporating fermented foods like sauerkraut or coconut yogurt can contribute to a balanced gut microbiome.

While the template provides structure, feel free to customize meals based on your preferences and dietary needs. Swap out protein sources, experiment with different vegetables, and rotate fats to keep meals exciting and satisfying.

By using meal templates, you streamline AIP meal planning, making it easier to create wholesome, flavorful dishes while adhering to the protocol's guidelines. Remember that individual needs may vary, so be attentive to your body's responses and work with a healthcare professional to fine-tune your AIP approach for optimal health and well-being.

8. STAY ORGANIZED: Keep a meal planning journal or digital document to record your weekly meal plans, recipes, and grocery lists. This helps you stay organized and avoid decision fatigue.

Staying organized is paramount when following the Autoimmune Protocol (AIP) to effectively manage conditions like Hashimoto's. Begin by creating a dedicated meal planning journal or digital document. Outline your weekly meal plans, jot down recipes, and compile comprehensive grocery lists. Consider batch cooking larger portions of AIP-friendly meals and freezing them for convenient, ready-to-eat options throughout the week. Label and date your freezer items to avoid confusion.

Set aside a specific day each week for meal prep, where you wash, chop, and portion out ingredients in advance. This proactive approach reduces cooking time on busier days and ensures AIP-compliant options are readily available. Invest in BPA-free food containers to keep prepared meals organized and easily accessible.

Moreover, clear out non-AIP foods from your pantry and fridge to minimize temptation and create a supportive environment. Label shelves or sections for AIP-approved ingredients, making it easy to locate items quickly. Keep a list of AIP-friendly snacks for on-the-go moments.

Tracking your progress is also essential for staying organized. Maintain a symptom journal to record changes in your health, energy levels, and any reactions to specific foods. Regularly consult this journal to assess the effectiveness of your AIP approach and make informed adjustments.

By establishing a structured routine, maintaining an organized kitchen, and diligently tracking your journey, you'll optimize your ability to adhere to the AIP and effectively manage Hashimoto's Thyroiditis, ultimately promoting a healthier and more balanced lifestyle.

9. LISTEN TO YOUR BODY: Pay attention to how your body responds to different foods and meals. Adjust your meal plans based on your individual needs and reactions.

Listening to your body is an essential practice when following the Autoimmune Protocol (AIP), especially when managing conditions like Hashimoto's Thyroiditis. AIP is a personalized approach, and tuning into your body's signals can guide you toward optimal health. Pay attention to how you feel after meals, noting any changes in energy levels, digestion, or symptoms. Keep a journal to track food reactions, mood fluctuations, and improvements. If certain foods elicit negative responses, eliminate or reintroduce them cautiously under professional guidance. Be patient and adaptable, as your body's responses may evolve over time. Prioritize rest, manage stress, and adjust your AIP plan as needed to maintain balance. Remember that everyone's journey is unique, and what works for one person may differ for another. By cultivating a mindful awareness of your body's cues, you empower yourself to make informed choices, tailor your AIP approach, and pave the way for better overall well-being and symptom management. Consulting a healthcare provider or registered dietitian can provide further insights and support as you navigate this healing journey.

By approaching AIP meal planning with dedication and enthusiasm, you can navigate the challenges of autoimmune management while enjoying a wide array of delicious and healthful dishes. Remember that becoming an AIP pro meal planner takes time and practice, so be patient with yourself as you develop your skills and create a sustainable routine that supports your well-being.

LOW-CARB MEAL PLAN

Creating a low-carb meal plan within the framework of the Autoimmune Protocol (AIP) requires careful selection of nutrient-dense, anti-inflammatory foods that comply with AIP guidelines. Here's a sample day of a low-carb AIP meal plan:

BREAKFAST:

- SCRAMBLED EGGS WITH SPINACH AND AVOCADO: Cook scrambled eggs with sautéed spinach in coconut oil. Serve with sliced avocado.

LUNCH:

- ROAST CHICKEN SALAD: Roast chicken breast over a bed of mixed greens, cucumbers, and radishes. Drizzle with olive oil and lemon juice.

SNACK:

- AIP-FRIENDLY BONE BROTH: Sip on a cup of homemade bone broth for a nourishing and low-carb snack.

DINNER:

- BAKED SALMON WITH CAULIFLOWER MASH: Bake salmon with lemon and dill. Prepare cauliflower mash by steaming cauliflower and mashing with coconut milk, garlic, and salt.

SNACK:

- SLICED TURKEY ROLL-UPS: Wrap turkey slices around carrot and cucumber sticks for a satisfying and crunchy snack.

NOTE: Keep in mind that AIP emphasizes nutrient density, so be sure to include a variety of non-starchy vegetables, healthy fats, and quality protein sources in each meal.

COCONUT FREE MEAL PLAN

Crafting a Coconut-Free AIP Meal Plan:
Nourishment and Flavor

For individuals navigating the Autoimmune
Protocol (AIP) while also avoiding coconut-based
products due to allergies or sensitivities, creating a
well-rounded and satisfying meal plan is not only
possible but can be a delightful culinary journey.
The AIP diet, designed to alleviate inflammation
and support healing, can still offer a diverse range
of flavors and nutrients without the inclusion of
coconut.

Breakfast:

Start your day with a nutrient-packed breakfast.
Opt for a vegetable-packed omelette cooked in
olive oil, filled with spinach, mushrooms, and
grated zucchini. Pair it with a side of sliced avocado
and a sprinkle of AIP-compliant herbs.

Lunch:

Prepare a refreshing salad with mixed greens,
grilled chicken or salmon, and a variety of colorful

vegetables like carrots, cucumbers, and bell peppers. Dress the salad with a tangy apple cider vinaigrette made from olive oil, apple cider vinegar, and AIP-approved herbs.

Snack:

Enjoy a handful of oven-baked sweet potato chips seasoned with a pinch of sea salt and rosemary. These satisfying and crunchy snacks are a perfect coconut-free option.

Dinner:

Indulge in a hearty dinner of roasted grass-fed beef or turkey served with a side of cauliflower mash. Steam broccoli and drizzle it with a lemon-garlic ghee sauce for a burst of flavor.

Dessert:

Satisfy your sweet tooth with baked cinnamon-spiced apples topped with a dollop of coconut-free coconut cream alternative or a dairy-free AIP-compliant ice cream.

Beverage:

Stay hydrated with herbal teas, infused water, or bone broth infused with aromatic herbs.

When crafting a coconut-free AIP meal plan, focus on incorporating nutrient-dense foods that support your healing journey while avoiding common allergens. Olive oil, avocado oil, and ghee can serve as excellent alternatives to coconut oil for cooking and flavor enhancement. Embrace the rich flavors of fresh herbs, quality meats, and an abundance of vegetables to create meals that are not only compliant with your dietary needs but also deeply satisfying to your palate. With creativity and careful planning, a coconut-free AIP meal plan can offer a diverse and nourishing culinary experience that promotes wellness and vitality.

EASY PEASY MEAL PLAN

Crafting an easy peasy meal plan for an Autoimmune Protocol (AIP) patient doesn't have to be daunting. With a focus on nutrient-dense foods that promote healing and minimize inflammation, here's a simple yet effective AIP meal plan that ensures convenience and nourishment.

Day 1:

Breakfast: Creamy coconut milk chia pudding topped with fresh berries and sliced toasted coconut.

Lunch: Grilled chicken salad with mixed greens, avocado, cucumber, and a homemade turmeric tahini dressing.

Dinner: Baked salmon with a side of steamed broccoli and sweet potato mash.

Day 2:

Breakfast: Smoothie with kale, avocado, frozen berries, coconut water, and collagen peptides.

Lunch: Zucchini noodles with cooked ground turkey, sautéed spinach, and a drizzle of olive oil.

- **Dinner:** Roasted chicken thighs seasoned with rosemary and garlic, alongside roasted carrots and a mixed greens salad.

Day 3:

- **Breakfast:** Sautéed kale and mushrooms with leftover roasted chicken, topped with a sprinkle of nutritional yeast.

Lunch: Tuna salad made with canned tuna, mixed greens, chopped cucumbers, and a lemon-ginger dressing.

Dinner: Beef stir-fry with colorful bell peppers, bok choy, and coconut aminos, served over cauliflower rice.

Day 4:

Breakfast: AIP-friendly apple-cinnamon muffins made with coconut flour and topped with coconut yogurt.

Lunch: Butternut squash soup with a side of sliced turkey roll-ups wrapped in lettuce leaves.

Dinner: Grilled pork chops with mashed sweet potatoes and a side of sautéed asparagus.

Day 5:

Breakfast: Sliced avocado topped with leftover salmon and a sprinkle of sea salt.

Lunch: Collard green wraps filled with leftover beef stir-fry and avocado slices.

Dinner: Baked cod with roasted Brussels sprouts and a side salad of mixed greens.

Snack Options: Sliced cucumber with guacamole, AIP-friendly beef jerky, carrot sticks with coconut yogurt dip.

Remember, preparation is key. Batch-cooking proteins, chopping vegetables, and having AIP-friendly condiments like turmeric tahini dressing or apple-cinnamon BBQ sauce on hand can make assembling meals a breeze. This easy peasy AIP meal plan showcases that with a bit of creativity and a focus on whole, nourishing ingredients, following the AIP diet can be both manageable and delicious.

ONE POT MEAL PLAN

Navigating the Autoimmune Protocol (AIP) diet can be a rewarding yet challenging journey, requiring meticulous planning and preparation. One-pot meals emerge as a saving grace, combining simplicity, nutrition, and taste. These meals not only streamline cooking but also adhere to AIP guidelines, eliminating potential trigger foods while keeping flavors diverse and wholesome. Here's a week-long one-pot meal plan for breakfast, lunch, and dinner, designed to support AIP patients in their healing process:

Breakfast:

Sweet Potato Hash: Start your day with a nutrient-packed sweet potato hash. Sauté diced sweet potatoes, ground turkey or pork, and a medley of colorful vegetables like bell peppers, onions, and spinach in coconut oil. Season with AIP-friendly herbs and spices like thyme and rosemary for a hearty breakfast that fuels your day.

Lunch:

Zucchini Noodle Bowl with Chicken: Prepare zucchini noodles using a spiralizer and cook them in a pot with olive oil. Add cooked shredded chicken, steamed broccoli, and a dollop of avocado pesto for a refreshing lunch. The combination of lean protein and veggies provides satiety and essential nutrients.

Dinner:

AIP-friendly Chili: Create a comforting one-pot chili using grass-fed ground beef, diced tomatoes, chopped carrots, and celery. Spice it up with turmeric, ginger, and garlic for flavor and anti-inflammatory benefits. Let it simmer and serve with a side of cauliflower rice for a fulfilling dinner.

Breakfast:

Baked Breakfast Casserole: Whisk together eggs, coconut milk, and AIP-approved veggies like kale, mushrooms, and butternut squash. Pour the mixture into a baking dish and bake until set. This hearty casserole can be sliced and reheated throughout the week.

Lunch:

Coconut Chicken Soup: Simmer bone broth, diced chicken, coconut milk, and an assortment of vegetables like carrots, bok choy, and zucchini in a single pot. Season with ginger, lemongrass, and

AIP-friendly herbs for a nourishing soup that's both soothing and satisfying.

Dinner:

Salmon and Asparagus Bake: Place wild-caught salmon fillets on a bed of asparagus spears in a baking dish. Drizzle with lemon juice, sprinkle with fresh dill, and bake until the salmon flakes easily. This simple yet elegant dish delivers omega-3 fatty acids and essential nutrients.

Breakfast:

Plantain Porridge: Cook sliced green plantains in coconut milk until softened. Mash them and top with sliced fruits, such as berries and kiwi, for added sweetness and antioxidants. A sprinkle of cinnamon rounds off this AIP-friendly breakfast option.

Lunch:

Cauliflower "Fried Rice": Pulse cauliflower florets in a food processor to create rice-like grains. Sauté with chopped AIP-friendly vegetables, diced chicken, and coconut aminos for a flavorful and satisfying lunch.

Dinner:

Turmeric Beef Stew: Brown grass-fed beef cubes in a pot, then add chopped root vegetables, such as carrots, parsnips, and turnips. Season with turmeric, thyme, and bay leaves, and let it simmer until tender. This warm stew is a perfect way to end the day.

By embracing the convenience and variety of one-pot meals, AIP patients can simplify their meal planning and preparation while adhering to their dietary needs. These recipes provide a balance of nutrients, flavors, and healing properties, supporting the journey towards better health and well-being. Remember, consulting a healthcare professional or nutritionist before making significant dietary changes is recommended, especially for those managing autoimmune conditions.

Comfort food meal plan

Following the Autoimmune Protocol (AIP) doesn't mean sacrificing delicious comfort foods. With careful planning and creativity, you can enjoy a week of comforting and healing meals that cater to your dietary needs. Here's a sample meal plan for a week, featuring AIP-friendly breakfast, lunch, and dinner options.

Day 1:

Breakfast: A warm bowl of "Noatmeal" made from mashed sweet potatoes, coconut milk, and a sprinkle of cinnamon. Top it with fresh berries and a drizzle of honey.

Lunch: Zucchini noodles with avocado pesto, cherry tomatoes, and grilled chicken. A side of mixed greens with a lemon-turmeric vinaigrette completes the meal.

Dinner: Slow-cooked beef stew with carrots, parsnips, and bone broth. Serve it with a side of mashed cauliflower and a sprinkle of chopped fresh parsley.

Day 2:

Breakfast: A smoothie bowl with blended coconut milk, frozen mixed berries, spinach, and collagen powder. Top with toasted coconut flakes and sliced kiwi.

Lunch: A lettuce wrap filled with tuna salad made with canned tuna, diced cucumbers, red onion, and avocado mayo. Enjoy it with a side of carrot sticks.

Dinner: Baked salmon fillet seasoned with dill and lemon, served with roasted Brussels sprouts and a sweet potato mash.

Day 3:

Breakfast: Sautéed kale and bacon topped with a poached egg. Pair with a side of sautéed mushrooms for added flavor.

Lunch: Butternut squash soup garnished with chopped chives and a drizzle of coconut cream. Enjoy with a mixed greens salad on the side.

Dinner: Grilled turkey burgers with lettuce, tomato, and onion wrapped in collard greens. Serve with a side of garlic roasted asparagus.

Day 4:

Breakfast: A coconut yogurt parfait layered with sliced bananas, toasted coconut, and a sprinkle of AIP-friendly granola.

Lunch: Roast chicken salad with mixed greens, roasted beets, shredded carrots, and a lemon-ginger dressing.

Dinner: Spaghetti squash with bolognese sauce made from ground beef, carrot, onion, and a tomato-free sauce. Sautéed spinach on the side adds an extra nutrient boost.

Day 5:

Breakfast: Baked apple halves stuffed with ground pork and cinnamon, topped with crushed toasted nuts.

Lunch: Collard green wraps filled with leftover bolognese sauce, sliced avocado, and julienned bell peppers.

Dinner: Herb-crusted pork chops with mashed cauliflower and a side of sautéed green beans.

Day 6:

Breakfast: Sautéed spinach and mushrooms with crispy AIP-friendly bacon.

Lunch: Chicken and vegetable stir-fry with coconut aminos, served over cauliflower rice.

Dinner: A hearty beef and vegetable stew slow-cooked for rich flavors. Accompany with a side of baked sweet potato fries.

Day 7:

Breakfast: A fruit salad with mixed berries, diced mango, and shredded coconut.

Lunch: A hearty avocado and mixed greens salad topped with leftover beef stew.

Dinner: Baked herbed chicken thighs with mashed parsnips and a side of steamed broccoli.

This sample meal plan showcases the diversity and creativity possible within the AIP guidelines, ensuring that comfort foods can be both satisfying and healing. Remember to adjust portion sizes and ingredients according to your personal preferences and dietary requirements.

Long-Term Maintenance and Beyond:

Navigating Long-Term Maintenance and Beyond with the Autoimmune Protocol (AIP)

Embarking on the Autoimmune Protocol (AIP) marks the beginning of a transformative journey towards better health and improved well-being. As you diligently follow the AIP guidelines and witness the positive changes it brings to your body and immune system, it's crucial to envision your path extending beyond the initial phases. Long-term maintenance is the next chapter in your AIP story, where sustainable habits and ongoing strategies become pivotal in maintaining the progress you've achieved and ensuring continued vitality.

The AIP, designed to identify and eliminate potential triggers that exacerbate autoimmune symptoms, serves as a comprehensive roadmap for healing. During the elimination phase, you've experienced the benefits of removing inflammatory foods, addressing gut health, and nurturing your body with nutrient-dense options. Now, transitioning to the long-term maintenance phase requires careful consideration of how to sustain these positive changes while gradually reintroducing certain foods to assess your individual tolerance levels.

Long-term maintenance involves three fundamental aspects:

1. Personalization: Throughout your AIP journey, you've gained insights into your body's responses and triggers. Leverage this knowledge to tailor your diet to your unique needs. While some individuals might find that certain reintroduced foods cause no adverse effects, others might discover sensitivities that require permanent avoidance. By personalizing your food choices, you can create a sustainable diet that nurtures your body and supports your health goals.

2. Reintroduction: Controlled and systematic reintroduction of eliminated foods is a crucial step in long-term maintenance. This process helps you identify which foods you can confidently incorporate back into your diet without causing inflammation or triggering autoimmune responses. The reintroduction phase demands patience and attention, as it involves testing one food group at a time and observing your body's reactions.

3. Holistic Lifestyle: Beyond dietary choices, holistic lifestyle factors play a pivotal role in long-term success. Adequate sleep, stress management, regular physical activity, and mindfulness contribute to overall well-being and immune

function. Integrate these practices into your daily routine to further support your health journey.

Embracing long-term maintenance with the AIP is not just about sustaining a specific diet but also about nurturing a lifestyle that promotes vitality, balance, and self-awareness. It's a commitment to self-care and a recognition of the power you hold in shaping your health trajectory. By acknowledging the ongoing nature of your journey and the evolving needs of your body, you set the stage for a life filled with wellness and resilience.

TRANSITIONING FROM ELIMINATION PHASE TO REINTRODUCTION

Navigating the transition from the elimination phase to the reintroduction phase of the Autoimmune Protocol (AIP) is a pivotal step in the journey towards understanding one's individual food sensitivities and crafting a sustainable, personalized dietary plan. The elimination phase, designed to reduce inflammation and allow the body to heal, involves temporarily removing potentially trigger foods. As this phase lays the foundation for healing, the reintroduction phase is the bridge that helps individuals identify which foods they can gradually reintroduce without triggering adverse reactions.

Transitioning to the reintroduction phase requires careful consideration and a systematic approach. Patience and mindfulness are key, as the primary goal is to observe how your body responds to the reintroduced foods. This phase enables you to discern which foods are well-tolerated and can be incorporated into your diet while avoiding those that may elicit symptoms.

Each individual's journey through reintroduction is unique, and factors such as symptom history, personal preferences, and health goals play a role in shaping this process. While it can be exciting to broaden your food choices, it's essential to proceed methodically and consult with a healthcare professional if needed. This transitional phase is not just about food; it's a voyage of self-discovery, empowerment, and fine-tuning your dietary choices to align with your health objectives. By approaching the reintroduction phase with mindfulness and dedication, you empower yourself to make informed decisions about the foods that support your well-being.

Sustainable Habits for Hashimoto's Remission

Embracing Sustainable Habits on the Path to Hashimoto's Remission with the AIP Diet

The journey towards achieving remission from Hashimoto's, an autoimmune disorder affecting the thyroid, demands more than just temporary changes in dietary habits. It necessitates a holistic and sustainable approach that extends beyond short-term fixes. The Autoimmune Protocol (AIP) offers a promising path to manage Hashimoto's symptoms and potentially achieve remission by focusing on inflammation reduction, immune system support, and gut health restoration. However, to truly experience lasting benefits, AIP patients must adopt sustainable habits that harmonize with their lifestyle and health goals.

Incorporating AIP principles into daily life involves more than adhering to a list of allowed and restricted foods. It's about cultivating a mindset shift towards nurturing the body, prioritizing self-care, and fostering long-term wellness. This requires a proactive approach to meal planning, sourcing quality ingredients, and practicing mindful eating. Equally vital is nurturing mental and emotional well-being, as stress management plays a pivotal role in autoimmune conditions.

In this exploration of sustainable habits for Hashimoto's remission within the framework of the AIP diet, we delve into actionable strategies that extend beyond dietary choices. From stress reduction techniques to fostering a supportive social network, we aim to empower AIP patients to not only manage their condition but also thrive. By embracing sustainable practices, individuals can embark on a transformative journey towards remission, optimizing their health and well-being for the long haul.

Preventing Flares and Sustaining Recovery with AIP

Navigating the journey of autoimmune conditions can be challenging, but the Autoimmune Protocol (AIP) offers a guiding light toward managing symptoms, preventing flares, and sustaining recovery. As individuals on this path, understanding the intricate relationship between diet and health is paramount. This guide aims to shed light on how AIP can serve as a powerful tool for maintaining wellness.

The AIP approach acknowledges the profound impact of certain foods on autoimmune responses, focusing on reducing inflammation and promoting gut health. By systematically eliminating potential trigger foods and incorporating nutrient-rich alternatives, AIP empowers individuals to take charge of their well-being. This guide will delve into the principles of the AIP framework, offering insights into selecting nourishing foods that support immune function, aid in healing, and prevent flares.

From crafting meals that cater to your body's unique needs to embracing lifestyle modifications that complement the dietary changes, this resource will provide you with actionable steps to create a sustainable and holistic approach to managing autoimmune conditions. By embracing AIP, you're embarking on a journey toward finding comfort, balance, and vitality while minimizing the impact of flares. Let's explore how the AIP approach can be your ally in preventing flares and fostering a lasting state of recovery.

www.ingramcontent.com/pod-product-compliance
Lightning Source LLC
Chambersburg PA
CBHW070820280726
48660CB00017B/2159